Delicious Plant Based Diet Cookbook 2021

Eat Healthy Food Learning Easy and Practical Plant Based Diet Recipes to Cook Every Day at Home, Losing Weight Fast

John Becker

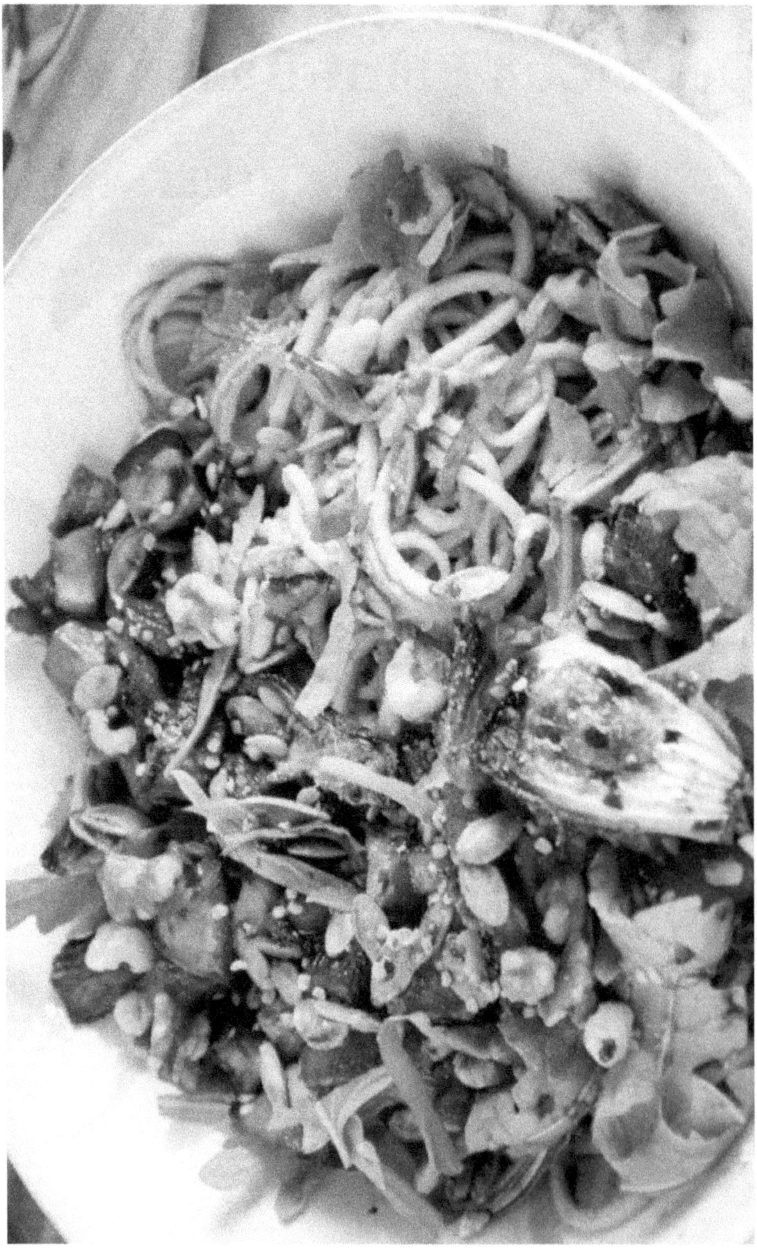

Table of Contents

The information in the following pages is broadly considered a truthful and accurate account of facts and as such, any inattention, use, or misuse of the information in question by the reader will render any resulting actions solely under their purview. There are no scenarios in which the publisher or the original author of this work can be in any fashion deemed liable for any hardship or damages that may befall them after undertaking information described herein.

Additionally, the information in the following pages is intended only for informational purposes and should thus be thought of as universal. As befitting its nature, it is presented without assurance regarding its prolonged validity or interim quality. Trademarks that are mentioned are done without written consent and can in no way be considered an endorsement from the trademark holder.

Introduction

A plant-based diet is a diet based primarily on whole plant foods. It is identical to the regular diet we're used to already, except that it leaves out foods that are not exclusively from plants. Hence, a plant-based diet does away with all types of animal-sourced foods, hydrogenated oils, refined sugars, and processed foods. A whole food plant-based diet comprises not just fruits and vegetables; it also consists of unprocessed or barely-processed oils with healthy monounsaturated fats (like extra-virgin olive oil), whole grains, legumes (essentially lentils and beans), seeds and nuts, as well as herbs and spices.

What makes a plant-based meal (or any meal) fun is the manner with which you make them; the seasoning process; and the combination process that contributes to a fantastic flavor and makes every meal unique and enjoyable. There are lots of delicious recipes (all plant-centered), which will prove helpful in when you intend making mouthwatering, healthy plant-based dishes for personal or household consumption. Provided you're eating these plant-based foods regularly, you'll have very problems with fat or diseases that result from bad dietary habits, and there would be no need for excessive calorie tracking.

Plant-based diet recipes are versatile; they range from colorful Salads to Lentil Stews, and Bean Burritos. The recipes also draw influences from around the globe, with Mexican, Chinese, European, Indian cuisines all part of the vast array of plant-based recipes available to choose from. Why You Ought to Reduce Your Intake of Processed and Animal-Based Foods. You have likely heard over and over that processed food has adverse effects on your health. You might have also been told repeatedly to stay away from foods with lots of preservatives; nevertheless, nobody ever offered any genuine or concrete facts about why you ought to avoid these foods and why they are unsafe. Consequently, let us properly dissect it to help you properly comprehend why you ought to stay away from these healthy eating offenders. They have massive habit-forming characteristics. Humans have a predisposition towards being addicted to some specific foods; however, the reality is that the fault is not wholly ours. Every one of the unhealthy treats we relish now and then triggers the dopamine release in our brains. This creates a pleasurable effect in our brain, but the excitement is usually short-lived. The discharged dopamine additionally causes an attachment connection gradually, and this is the reason some people consistently go back to eat certain unhealthy foods even when they know it's unhealthy and unnecessary. You can get rid of this by taking out that inducement completely. They are sugar-laden and plenteous in glucose-fructose syrup. Animal-based and processed foods are laden with refined sugars and glucose-fructose syrup which has almost no beneficial food nutrient. An ever-increasing number of studies are affirming what several people presumed from the start; that genetically modified foods bring about inflammatory bowel disease, which consequently makes it increasingly difficult for the body to assimilate essential nutrients. The disadvantages that result from your body being unable to assimilate essential nutrients from consumed foods rightly cannot be overemphasized. Processed and animal-based food products contain plenteous amounts of refined carbohydrates. Indeed, your body requires carbohydrates to give it the needed energy to run body capacities. In any case, refining carbs dispenses with the fundamental supplements; in the way that refining entire grains disposes of the whole grain part. What remains, in the wake of refining, is what's considered as empty carbs or empty calories. These can negatively affect the metabolic system in your body by sharply increasing your blood sugar and insulin quantities. They contain lots of synthetic

—

ingredients. At the point when your body is taking in non-natural ingredients, it regards them as foreign substances. Your body treats them as a health threat. Your body isn't accustomed to identifying synthetic compounds like sucralose or these synthesized sugars. Hence, in defense of your health against this foreign "aggressor," your body does what it's capable of to safeguard your health. It sets off an immune reaction to tackle this "enemy" compound, which indirectly weakens your body's general disease alertness, making you susceptible to illnesses. The concentration and energy expended by your body in ensuring your immune system remain safe could instead be devoted somewhere else. They contain constituent elements that set off an excitable reward sensation in your body. A part of processed and animal-based foods contain compounds like glucose-fructose syrup, monosodium glutamate, and specific food dyes that can trigger some addiction. They rouse your body to receive a benefit in return whenever you consume them. Monosodium glutamate, for example, is added to many store-bought baked foods. This additive slowly conditions your palates to relish the taste. It gets mental just by how your brain interrelates with your taste sensors.

This reward-centric arrangement makes you crave it increasingly, which ends up exposing you to the danger of over consuming calories.

For animal protein, usually, the expression "subpar" is used to allude to plant proteins since they generally have lower levels of essential amino acids as against animal-sourced protein. Nevertheless, what the vast majority don't know is that large amounts of essential amino acids can prove detrimental to your health. Let me break it down further for you.

Veggie Noodles

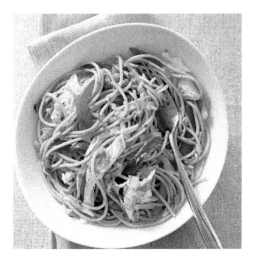

Preparation Time: 10 Minutes

Cooking Time: 5 Minutes

Serving: 2

Ingredients:

- 2 tablespoons vegetable oil
- 4 spring onions, divided
- 1 cup snap pea
- 2 tablespoons brown sugar
- 9 oz. dried rice noodles, cooked
- 5 garlic cloves, minced
- 2 carrots, cut into small sticks
- 3 tablespoons soy sauce

Directions:

Heat vegetable oil in a skillet over medium heat and
add garlic and 3 spring onions.

Cook for about 3 minutes and add the carrots, peas,
brown sugar and soy sauce.

Add rice noodles and cook for about 2 minutes.

Season with salt and black pepper and top with
remaining spring onion to serve.

Nutrition:

Calories: 411

Net Carbs: 47.3g

Fat: 14.3g

Carbohydrates: 63.6g

Fiber: 7.6g

Sugar: 17g

Protein: 8.1g

Sodium: 1431mg

5 Ingredients Pasta

Preparation Time: 15 minutes

Cooking Time: 25 minutes

Servings: 5

Ingredients:

1 (25 oz.) jar marinara sauce

Olive oil, as needed

1 pound dry vegan pasta

1 pound assorted vegetables, like red onion, zucchini and
tomatoes

¼ cup prepared hummus

Salt, to taste

Directions:

Preheat the oven to 400 degrees F and grease a large baking
sheet.

Arrange the vegetables in a single layer on the baking sheet
and sprinkle with olive oil and salt.

Transfer into the oven and roast the vegetables for about 15
minutes.

Boil salted water in a large pot and cook the pasta according
to the package directions.

Drain the water when the pasta is tender and put the pasta
in a colander.

Mix together the marinara sauce and hummus in a large pot to make a creamy sauce.

Stir in the cooked vegetables and pasta to the sauce and toss to coat well.

Dish out in a bowl and serve warm.

NUTRITION:

Calories: 415

Total Fat: 29g

Protein: 33g

Total Carbs: 5.5g

Fiber: 2g

Net Carbs: 3.5g

Dip and Spread Recipes

Asparagus Spanakopita

Preparation Time: 25 minutes

Cooking Time: 25 minutes

Servings: 12

Ingredients:

- 2 cups cut fresh asparagus (1-inch pieces)
- 20 sheets phyllo dough, (14 inches x 9 inches)
- Nonstick cooking spray
- Refrigerated butter-flavored spray
- 2 cups torn fresh spinach
- 3 oz. crumbled feta cheese
- 2 tablespoon vegan butter
- 1/4 cup all-purpose flour
- 1-1/2 cups Fat-free milk
- 3 tablespoon lemon juice
- 1 teaspoon dill weed
- 1 teaspoon dried thyme
- 1/4 teaspoon salt

Directions:

1. In a steamer basket, put the asparagus and place it on top of a saucepan with 1-inch of water, then boil. Put the cover and let it steam for 5 minutes or until it becomes crisp-tender.

2. Put 1 sheet of phyllo dough in a cooking spray-coated 13x9-inch baking dish, then cut if needed. Use the butter-flavored spray to spritz the dough. Redo the layers 9 times. Lay the asparagus, feta cheese, and spinach on top. Cover it using a sheet of phyllo dough, then spritz it using the butter-flavored spray. Redo the process using the leftover phyllo. Slice it into 12 pieces. Let it bake for 15 minutes at 350 degrees F without cover, or until it turns golden brown.

3. To make the sauce, in a small saucepan, melt the butter. Mix in the flour until it becomes smooth, then slowly add the milk. Stir in salt, thyme, dill, and lemon juice, then boil. Let it cook and stir for 5 minutes until it becomes thick. Serve the spanakopita with the sauce.

Nutrition:

Calories 112,Fat 4,Carbs 14,Protein 5

Black Bean and Corn Salsa from Red Gold

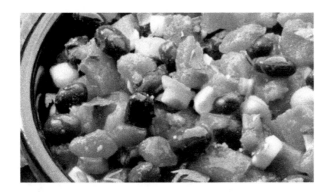

Preparation Time: 15 minutes

Cooking Time: 15 minutes

Servings: 25

Ingredients:

- 2 cans black beans, drained and rinsed
- 1 can whole kernel corn, drained
- 2 cans RED GOLD® Petite Diced Tomatoes & Green Chilies
- 1 can RED GOLD® Diced Tomatoes, drained
- 1/2 cup chopped green onions
- 2 tablespoon chopped fresh cilantro
- Salt and black pepper to taste

Directions:

1. Mix all ingredients to combine in a big bowl. Refrigerate to blend flavors for a few hours to overnight. Serve with chips or crackers.

Nutrition:

Calories 65

Fat 3

Carbs 8

Protein 9

Avocado Bean Dip

Preparation Time: 15 minutes

Cooking Time: 15 minutes

Servings: 2

Ingredients:

> 1 medium ripe avocado, peeled and cubed
>
> 1/2 cup fresh cilantro leaves
>
> 3 tablespoon lime juice
>
> 1/2 teaspoon onion powder
>
> 1/2 teaspoon garlic powder
>
> 1/2 teaspoon chipotle hot pepper sauce
>
> 1/4 teaspoon salt
>
> 1/4 teaspoon ground cumin
>
> Baked tortilla chips

Directions:

> Mix the first 9 ingredients in a food processor, then cover and blend until smooth. Serve along with chips.

Nutrition:

Calories 85

Fat 4

Carbs 13

Protein 6

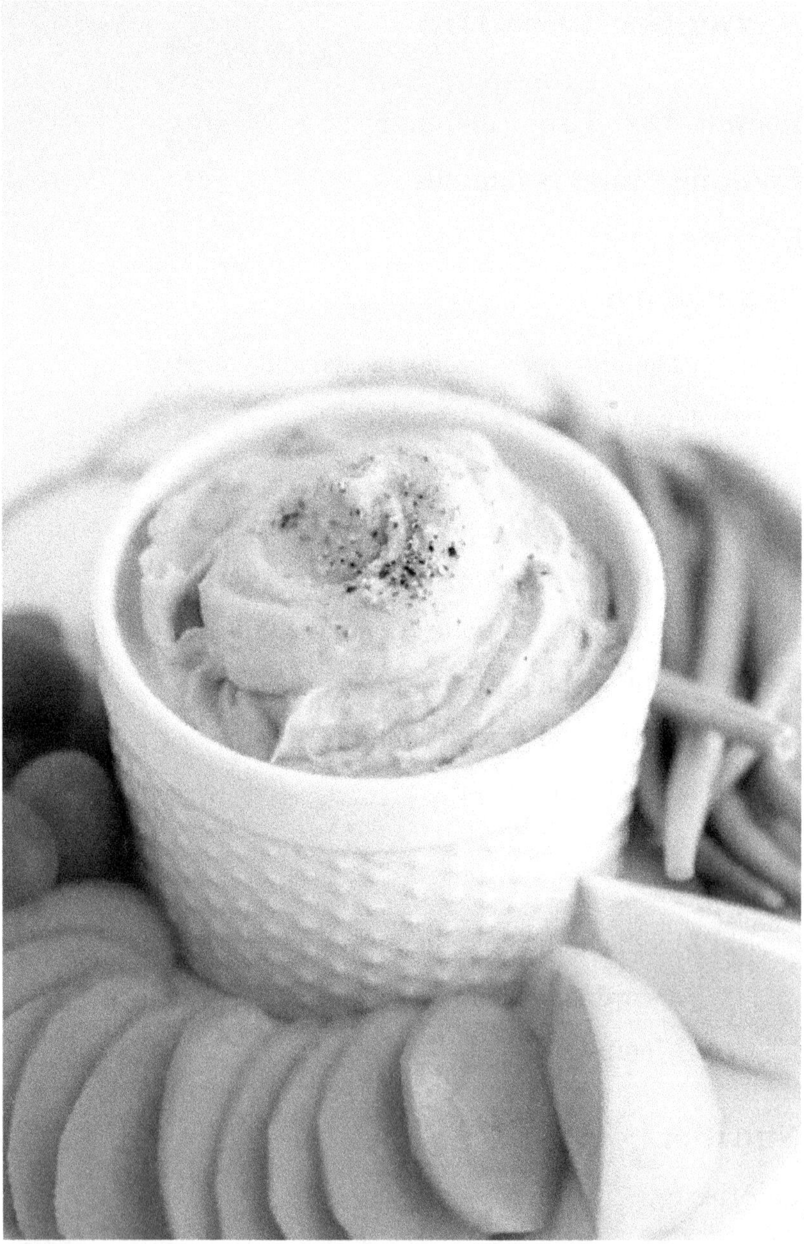

Crunchy Peanut Butter Apple Dip

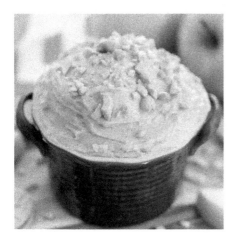

Preparation Time: 10 minutes

Cooking Time: 10 minutes

Servings: 2

Ingredients:

  1 carton (8 oz.) reduced-Fat spreadable cream cheese

  1 cup creamy peanut butter

  1/4 cup Fat-free milk

  1 tablespoon brown sugar

  1 teaspoon vanilla extract

  1/2 cup chopped unsalted peanuts

  Apple slices

Directions:

Beat the initial 5 ingredients in a small bowl until combined. Mix in peanuts. Serve with slices of apple, then put the leftovers in the fridge.

Nutrition:

Calories 125

Fat 5

Carbs 23

Protein 9

Herb Pockets

Preparation Time: 25 minutes

Cooking Time: 25 minutes

Servings: 3

Ingredients:

2/3 cup reduced-Fat garlic-herb spreadable cheese

4 oz. reduced-Fat cream cheese

2 tablespoon half-and-half cream

1 garlic clove, minced

1 tablespoon dried basil

1 teaspoon dried thyme

1/2 teaspoon celery salt

1/4 teaspoon dill weed

1/4 teaspoon salt

1/4 teaspoon pepper

3 to 4 drops hot pepper sauce

1/2 cup chopped canned water-packed artichoke
   hearts, rinsed and drained

1/4 cup chopped roasted red peppers

2 tubes (8 oz. each) refrigerated reduced-Fat crescent
   rolls

Directions:

Beat garlic, cream, cream cheese, and spreadable
cheese until blended in a small bowl. Beat in hot
pepper sauce, pepper, salt, and herbs. Fold in red
peppers and artichokes. Refrigerate, covered, for at
least an hour.

Unroll both crescent roll dough tubes. Form every
dough tube to a long rectangle on a lightly floured
surface. Seal perforations and seams. Roll each to a
16x12-in. rectangle. Cut to 4 strips, lengthwise and
3 strips, width wise. Separate squares.

In the middle of each square, put 1 rounded tablespoon
filling. Fold into half, making triangles. Seal by
crimping edges. Trim if needed. Put onto ungreased
baking sheets. Bake for 10-15 minutes or until
golden brown at 375 degrees F. Serve warm.

Nutrition:

Calories 245

Fat 5

Carbs 10

Protein 7

Creamy Cucumber Yogurt Dip

Preparation Time: 15 minutes

Cooking Time: 15 minutes

Servings: 4

Ingredients:

1 cup (8 oz.) reduced-Fat plain yogurt

4 oz. reduced-Fat cream cheese

1/2 cup chopped seeded peeled cucumber

1-1/2 teaspoon. finely chopped onion

1-1/2 teaspoon. Snipped fresh dill or 1/2 teaspoon dill
weed

1 teaspoon lemon juice

1 teaspoon grated lemon peel

1 garlic clove, minced

1/4 teaspoon salt

1/4 teaspoon pepper

Assorted fresh vegetables

Directions:

Mix the cream cheese and yogurt in a small bowl. Stir
in pepper, salt, garlic, peel, lemon juice, dill, onion,
and cucumber. Put on the cover and let it chill in
the fridge. Serve it with the veggies.

Nutrition:

Calories 55

Fat 4

Carbs 12

Protein 6

Chunky Cucumber Salsa

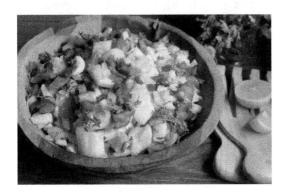

Preparation Time: 20 minutes

Cooking Time: 20 minutes

Servings: 4

Ingredients:

 3 medium cucumbers, peeled and coarsely chopped

 1 medium mango, coarsely chopped

 1 cup frozen corn, thawed

 1 medium sweet red pepper, coarsely chopped

 1 small red onion, coarsely chopped

 1 jalapeno pepper, finely chopped

 3 garlic cloves, minced

 2 tablespoon white wine vinegar

 1 tablespoon minced fresh cilantro

 1 teaspoon salt

 1/2 teaspoon sugar

 1/4 to 1/2 teaspoon cayenne pepper

Directions:

Mix all ingredients in a big bowl, then chill, covered, about 2 to 3 hours before serving.

Nutrition:

Calories 215

Fat 5

Carbs 23

Protein 10

Healthier Guacamole

Preparation Time: 10 minutes

Cooking Time: 10 minutes

Servings: 4

Ingredients:

> 3/4 cup crumbled tofu
>
> 2 avocados - peeled and pitted, divided
>
> 1 teaspoon salt
>
> 1 teaspoon minced garlic
>
> 1 pinch cayenne pepper (optional)

Directions:

Prepare a food processor then put one avocado and
   tofu in it then blend well until it becomes smooth.
   Combine salt, lime juice, and the left avocado in a
   bowl.

Add in the garlic, tomatoes, cilantro, onion, and tofu-
   avocado mixture. Put in cayenne pepper.

Let it chill in the refrigerator for 1 hour to enhance the
   flavor or you can serve it right away.

Nutrition:

Calories 534,Fat 5,Carbs 23,Protein 11

Garlic White Bean Dip

Preparation Time: 15 minutes

Cooking Time: 15 minutes

Servings: 2

Ingredients:

1/4 cup soft bread crumbs

2 tablespoon dry white wine or water

2 tablespoon olive oil

2 tablespoon lemon juice

4-1/2 teaspoon. Minced fresh parsley

3 garlic cloves, peeled and halved

1/2 teaspoon salt

1/2 teaspoon snipped fresh dill or 1/4 teaspoon dill
weed

1/8 teaspoon cayenne pepper

Assorted fresh vegetables

Directions:

Mix wine and bread crumbs in a small bowl. Mix
cayenne, dill, salt, garlic, parsley, beans, lemon
juice, and oil in a food processor, then cover and
blend until smooth.

Put in bread crumb mixture and process until well
combined. Serve together with vegetables.

Nutrition:

Calories 105

Fat 5

Carbs 12

Protein 6

Fruit Skewers

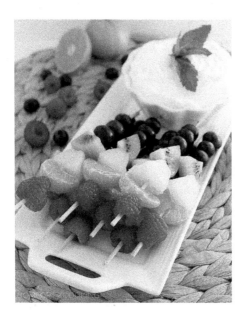

Preparation Time: 20 minutes

Cooking Time: 20 minutes

Servings: 2

Ingredients:

Cream cheese

Fat sour cream

Lime juice

Honey

1/2 teaspoon ground ginger

2 cups green grapes

2 cups fresh or canned unsweetened pineapple chunks

2 large red apples, cut into 1-inch pieces

Directions:

To make the dip, beat the sour cream and cream cheese in a small bowl until it becomes smooth. Beat in the ginger, honey, and lime juice until it becomes smooth.

Put the cover and let it chill in the fridge for a minimum of 1 hour.

Alternately thread the apples, pineapple, and grapes on 8 12-inch skewers. Serve it right away with the dip.

Nutrition:

Calories 180

Fat 5

Carbs 28

Protein 4

Light & Creamy Garlic Hummus

Preparation Time: 10 minutes

Cooking Time: 40 minutes

Servings: 12

Ingredients:

- 1 1/2 cups dry chickpeas, rinsed

- 2 1/2 tbsp. fresh lemon juice

- 1 tbsp. garlic, minced

- 1/2 cup tahini

- cups of water

Directions

- Add water and chickpeas into the instant pot.

- Seal pot with a lid and select manual and set timer for 40 minutes.

- Once done, allow to release pressure naturally. Remove lid.

- Drain chickpeas well and reserved 1/2 cup chickpeas liquid.

- Transfer chickpeas, reserved liquid, lemon juice, garlic, tahini, pepper, and salt into the food processor and process until smooth.

- Serve and enjoy.

Nutrition: 152 Calories 6.9g Fat 17g Carbohydrates

Marinated Mushrooms

Preparation Time: 15 minutes

Cooking Time: 25 minutes

Servings: 8

Ingredients:

1 cup red wine

1/2 cup red wine vinegar

1/3 cup olive oil

2 tablespoon brown sugar

2 cloves garlic, minced

1 teaspoon crushed red pepper flakes

1/4 cup red bell pepper, diced

1 lb. small fresh mushrooms, washed and trimmed

1/4 cup chopped green onions

1/4 teaspoon dried oregano

1/2 teaspoon salt

1/4 teaspoon ground black pepper

Directions:

Mix the mushrooms, red pepper flakes, bell pepper, garlic, sugar, oil, vinegar, and wine in a saucepan on medium heat, then boil.

Put the cover and put it aside to let it cool.

Mix in pepper, salt, oregano, and green onions once cooled. Serve it at room temperature or chilled.

Nutrition:

Calories 135

Fat 5

Carbs 13

Protein 8

Pumpkin Spice Spread

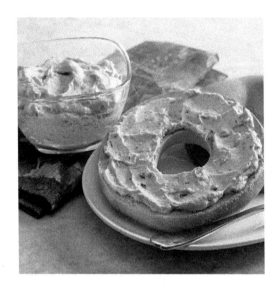

Preparation Time: 10 minutes

Cooking Time: 10 minutes

Servings: 4

Ingredients:

> 1 package (8 oz.) Fat-free cream cheese
>
> 1/2 cup canned pumpkin
>
> Sugar substitute equivalent to 1/2 cup sugar
>
> 1 teaspoon ground cinnamon
>
> 1 teaspoon vanilla extract
>
> 1 teaspoon maple flavoring
>
> 1/2 teaspoon pumpkin pie spice

1/2 teaspoon ground nutmeg

1 carton (8 oz.) frozen reduced-Fat whipped topping, thawed

Directions:

Mix well together sugar substitute, pumpkin, and cream cheese in a big bowl. Beat in nutmeg, pumpkin pie spice, maple flavoring, vanilla, and cinnamon.

Fold in whipped topping and chill until serving.

Nutrition:

Calories 177

Fat 6

Carbs 21

Protein 11

Maple Bagel Spread

Preparation Time: 10 minutes

Cooking Time: 10 minutes

Servings: 1

Ingredients:

> cream cheese
>
> maple syrup
>
> cinnamon
>
> walnuts

Directions:

> Beat the cinnamon, syrup, and cream cheese in a big
>> bowl until it becomes smooth, then mix in walnuts.
>
> Let it chill until ready to serve. Serve it with bagels.

Nutrition:

Calories 586

Fat 7

Carbs 23

Protein 4

Italian Stuffed Artichokes

Preparation Time: 20 minutes

Cooking Time: 25 minutes

Servings: 4

Ingredients:

4 large artichokes

2 teaspoon lemon juice

2 cups soft Italian bread crumbs, toasted

1/2 cup grated Parmigiano-Reggiano cheese

1/2 cup minced fresh parsley

2 teaspoon Italian seasoning

1 teaspoon grated lemon peel

1/2 teaspoon pepper

1/4 teaspoon salt

1 tablespoon olive oil

Directions:

Level the bottom of each artichoke using a sharp knife and trim off 1-inch from the tops. Snip off tips of outer leaves using kitchen scissors, then brush lemon juice on cut edges. In a Dutch oven, stand the artichokes and pour 1-inch of water, then boil. Lower the heat, put the cover, and let it simmer for 5 minutes or until the leaves near the middle pull out effortlessly.

Turn the artichokes upside down to drain. Allow it to stand for 10 minutes. Carefully scrape out the fuzzy middle part of the artichokes using a spoon and get rid of it.

Mix the salt, pepper, lemon peel, Italian seasoning, garlic, parsley, cheese, and breadcrumbs in a small bowl, then add olive oil and stir well. Gently spread the artichoke leaves apart, then fill it with breadcrumb mixture.

Put it in a cooking spray-coated 11x7-inch baking dish. Let it bake for 10 minutes at 350 degrees F without cover, or until the filling turns light brown.

Nutrition:

Calories 543

Fat 5

Carbs 44

Protein 6

Enchilada sauce

Preparation Time: 10 minutes

Cooking Time: 10 minutes

Servings: 13

Ingredients:

> 1½ tablespoon MCT oil
>
> ½ tablespoon chili powder
>
> ½ tablespoon whole wheat flour
>
> ½ teaspoon ground cumin
>
> ¼ teaspoon oregano (dried or fresh)
>
> ¼ teaspoon salt (or to taste)
>
> 1 garlic clove (minced)
>
> 1 tablespoon tomato paste
>
> 1 cup vegetable broth
>
> ½ teaspoon apple vinegar
>
> ½ teaspoon ground black pepper

Directions:

Heat a small saucepan over medium heat.

Add the MCT oil and minced garlic to the pan and sauté for about 1 minute.

Mix the dry spices and flour in a medium bowl and pour the dry mixture into the saucepan.

Stir in the tomato paste immediately, and slowly pour
in the vegetable broth, making sure that everything
combines well.

When everything is mixed thoroughly, bring up the
heat to medium-high until it gets to a simmer and
cook for about 3 minutes or until the sauce
becomes a bit thicker.

Remove the pan from the heat and add the vinegar
with the black pepper, adding more salt and pepper
to taste.

Nutrition:

Calories 225

Fat 4

Carbs 33

Protein 5

Vegetables Recipes

Crusty Grilled Corn

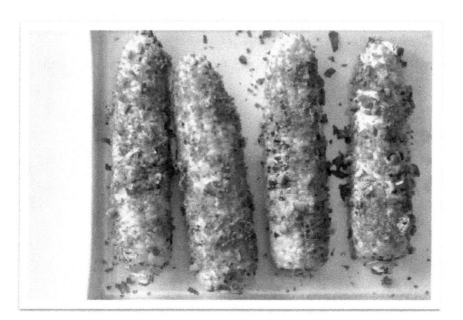

Preparation Time: 10 minutes

Cooking Time: 15 minutes

Servings: 4

Ingredients:

- 2 corn cobs
- 1/3 cup Vegenaise
- 1 small handful cilantro

- ½ cup breadcrumbs
- 1 teaspoon lemon juice

Directions:

2. Preheat the gas grill on high heat.
3. Add corn grill to the grill and continue grilling until it turns golden-brown on all sides.
4. Mix the Vegenaise, cilantro, breadcrumbs, and lemon juice in a bowl.
5. Add grilled corn cobs to the crumbs mixture.
6. Toss well then serve.

Nutrition:

Calories: 253

Total Fat: 13g

Protein: 31g

Total Carbs: 3g

Fiber: 0g

Net Carbs: 3g

Grilled Carrots with Chickpea Salad

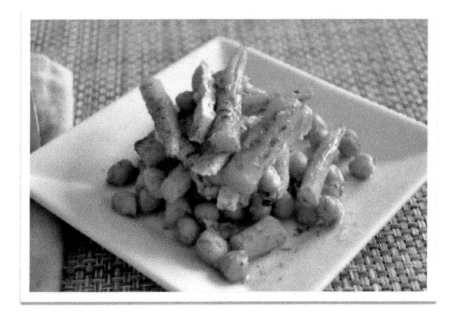

Preparation Time: 10 minutes

Cooking Time: 10 minutes

Servings: 8

Ingredients:

- Carrots

- 8 large carrots
- 1 tablespoon oil
- 1 ½ teaspoon salt
- 1 teaspoon dried oregano

- 1 teaspoon dried thyme
- 2 teaspoon paprika powder
- 1 ½ tablespoon soy sauce
- ½ cup of water
- Chickpea Salad
- 14 oz canned chickpeas
- 3 medium pickles
- 1 small onion
- A big handful of lettuce
- 1 teaspoon apple cider vinegar
- ½ teaspoon dried oregano
- ½ teaspoon salt
- Ground black pepper, to taste
- ½ cup vegan cream

Directions:

- Toss the carrots with all of its ingredients in a bowl.
- Thread one carrot on a stick and place it on a plate.
- Preheat the grill over high heat.
- Grill the carrots for 2 minutes per side on the grill.
- Toss the ingredients for the salad in a large salad bowl.

- Slice grilled carrots and add them on top of the salad.
- Serve fresh.

Nutrition:

Calories: 661

Total Fat: 68g

Carbs: 17g

Net Carbs: 7g

Fiber: 2g

Protein: 4g

Grilled Avocado Guacamole

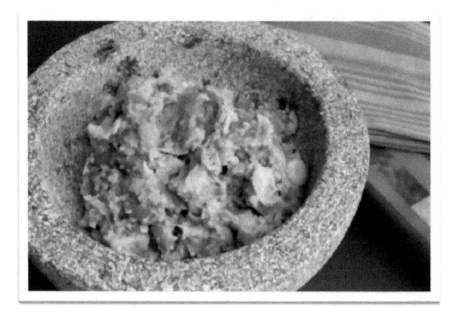

Preparation Time: 10 minutes

Cooking Time: 20 minutes

Servings: 4

Ingredients:

- ½ teaspoon olive oil
- 1 lime, halved
- ½ onion, halved
- 1 serrano chile, halved, stemmed, and seeded
- 3 Haas avocados, skin on
- 2–3 tablespoons fresh cilantro, chopped
- ½ teaspoon smoked salt

Directions:

1. Preheat the grill over medium heat.
2. Brush the grilling grates with olive oil and place chile, onion, and lime on it.
3. Grill the onion for 10 minutes, chile for 5 minutes, and lime for 2 minutes.
4. Transfer the veggies to a large bowl.
5. Now cut the avocados in half and grill them for 5 minutes.
6. Mash the flesh of the grilled avocado in a bowl.
7. Chop the other grilled veggies and add them to the avocado mash.
8. Stir in remaining ingredients and mix well.
9. Serve.

Nutrition:

Calories: 165

Total Fat: 17g

Carbs: 4g

Net Carbs: 2g

Fiber: 1g

Protein: 1g

Grilled Fajitas with Jalapeño Sauce

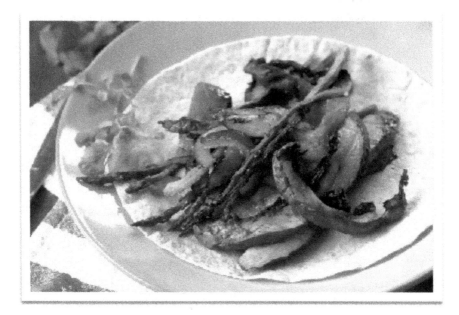

Preparation Time: 10 minutes

Cooking Time: 25 minutes

Servings: 4

Ingredients:

Marinade

¼ cup olive oil

¼ cup lime juice

2 garlic cloves, minced

1 teaspoon chili powder

1 teaspoon ground cumin

1 teaspoon dried oregano

½ teaspoon salt

½ teaspoon black pepper

Jalapeño Sauce

6 jalapeno peppers stemmed, halved, and seeded

1–2 teaspoons olive oil

1 cup raw cashews, soaked and drained

½ cup almond milk

¼ cup water

¼ cup lime juice

2 teaspoons agaves

½ cup fresh cilantro

Salt, to taste

Grilled Vegetables

½ lb asparagus spears, trimmed

2 large portobello mushrooms, sliced

1 large zucchini, sliced

1 red bell pepper, sliced

1 red onion, sliced

Directions:

Dump all the ingredients for the marinade in a large bowl.

Toss in all the veggies and mix well to marinate for 1 hour.

Meanwhile, prepare the sauce and brush the jalapenos with
  oil.

Grill the jalapenos for 5 minutes per side until slightly
  charred.

Blend the grilled jalapenos with other ingredients for the
sauce in a blender.

Transfer this sauce to a separate bowl and keep it aside.

Now grill the marinated veggies in the grill until soft and
slightly charred on all sides.

Pour the prepared sauce over the grilled veggies.

Serve.

Nutrition:

Calories: 663

Total Fat: 68g

Carbs: 20g

Net Carbs: 10g

Fiber: 2g

Protein: 4g

Grilled Ratatouille Kebabs

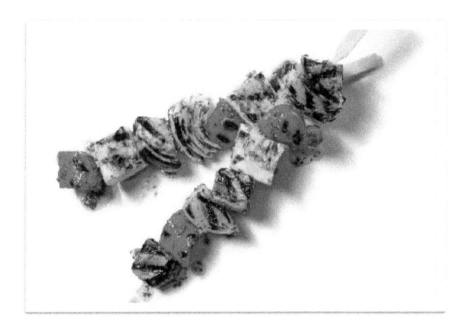

Preparation Time: 10 minutes

Cooking Time: 20 minutes

Servings: 6

Ingredients:

   3 tablespoons soy sauce

   3 tablespoons balsamic vinegar

   1 teaspoon dried thyme leaves

   2 tablespoons extra virgin olive oil

   Veggies

   1 zucchini, diced

   ½ red onion, diced

½ red capsicum, diced

2 tomatoes, diced

1 small eggplant, diced

8 button mushrooms, diced

Directions:

Toss the veggies with soy sauce, olive oil, thyme, and balsamic vinegar in a large bowl.

Thread the veggies alternately on the wooden skewers and reserve the remaining marinade.

Marinate these skewers for 1 hour in the refrigerator.

Preheat the grill over medium heat.

Grill the marinated skewers for 5 minutes per side while basting with the reserved marinade.

Serve fresh.

Nutrition:

Calories: 166

Total Fat: 17g

Carbs: 5g

Net Carbs: 3g

Fiber: 1g

Protein: 1g

Tofu Hoagie Rolls

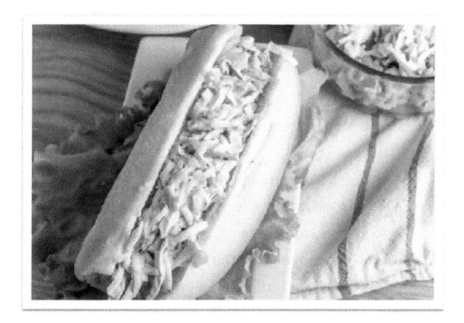

Preparation Time: 10 minutes

Cooking Time: 20 minutes

Servings: 6

Ingredients:

½ cup vegetable broth

¼ cup hot sauce

1 tablespoon vegan butter

1 (16 ounce) package tofu, pressed and diced

4 cups cabbage, shredded

2 medium apples, grated

1 medium shallot, grated

6 tablespoons vegan mayonnaise

1 tablespoon apple cider vinegar

Salt and black pepper

4 6-inch hoagie rolls, toasted

Directions:

In a saucepan, combine broth with butter and hot sauce and
bring to a boil.

Add tofu and reduce the heat to a simmer.

Cook for 10 minutes then remove from heat and let sit for
10 minutes to marinate.

Toss cabbage and rest of the ingredients in a salad bowl.

Prepare and set up a grill on medium heat.

Drain the tofu and grill for 5 minutes per side.

Lay out the toasted hoagie rolls and add grilled tofu to each
hoagie

Add the cabbage mixture evenly between them then close it.

Serve.

Nutrition:

Calories: 111

Total Fat: 11g

Carbs: 5g

Net Carbs: 1g

Fiber: 0g

Protein: 1g

Grilled Avocado with Tomatoes

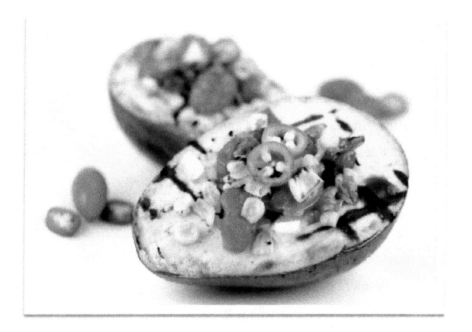

Preparation Time: 10 minutes

Cooking Time: 15 minutes

Servings: 6

Ingredients:

3 avocados, halved and pitted

3 limes, wedged

1½ cup grape tomatoes

1 cup fresh corn

1 cup onion, chopped

3 serrano peppers

2 garlic cloves, peeled

¼ cup cilantro leaves, chopped

1 tablespoon olive oil

Salt and black pepper to taste

Directions:

Prepare and set a grill over medium heat.

Brush the avocado with oil and grill it for 5 minutes per side.

Meanwhile, toss the garlic, onion, corn, tomatoes, and pepper in a baking sheet.

At 550 degrees F, roast the vegetables for 5 minutes.

Toss the veggie mix and stir in salt, cilantro, and black pepper.

Mix well then fill the grilled avocadoes with the mixture.

Garnish with lime.

Serve.

Nutrition:

Calories: 56

Total Fat: 6g

Carbs: 3g

Net Carbs: 1g

Fiber: 0g

Protein: 1g

Grilled Tofu with Chimichurri Sauce

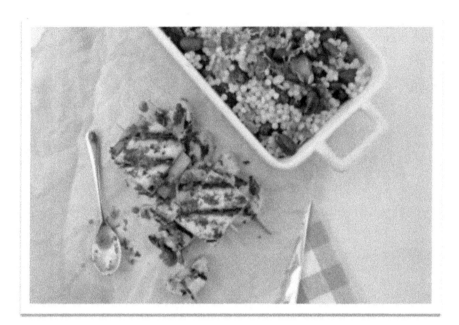

Preparation Time: 10 minutes

Cooking Time: 12 minutes

Servings: 4

Ingredients:

- 2 tablespoons plus 1 teaspoon olive oil
- 1 teaspoon dried oregano
- 1 cup parsley leaves
- ½ cup cilantro leaves
- 2 Fresno peppers, seeded and chopped
- 2 tablespoons white wine vinegar
- 2 tablespoons water

1 tablespoon fresh lime juice

Salt and black pepper

1 cup couscous, cooked

1 teaspoon lime zest

¼ cup toasted pumpkin seeds

1 cup fresh spinach, chopped

1 (15.5 ounce) can kidney beans, rinsed and drained

1 (14 to 16 ounce) block tofu, diced

2 summer squashes, diced

3 spring onions, quartered

Directions:

In a saucepan, heat 2 tablespoons oil and add oregano over
medium heat.

After 30 seconds add parsley, chili pepper, cilantro, lime
juice, 2 tablespoons water, vinegar, salt and black
pepper.

Mix well then blend in a blender.

Add the remining oil, pumpkin seeds, beans and spinach
and cook for 3 minutes.

Stir in couscous and adjust seasoning with salt and black
pepper.

Prepare and set up a grill on medium heat.

Thread the tofu, squash, and onions on the skewer in an
alternating pattern.

Grill these skewers for 4 minutes per side while basting
with the green sauce.

Serve the skewers on top of the couscous with green sauce.
Enjoy.

Nutrition:

Calories: 813

Total Fat: 83g

Carbs: 25g

Net Carbs: 11g

Fiber: 1g

Protein: 7g

Grilled Seitan with Creole Sauce

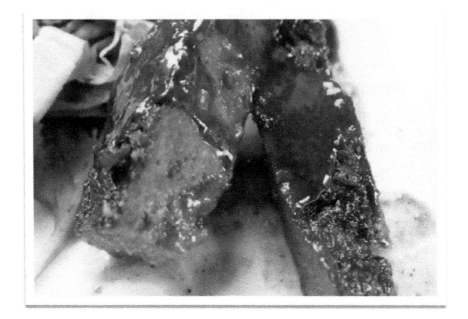

Preparation Time: 10 minutes

Cooking Time: 14 minutes

Servings: 4

Ingredients:

Grilled Seitan Kebabs:

    4 cups seitan, diced

    2 medium onions, diced into squares

    8 bamboo skewers

    1 can coconut milk

    2½ tablespoons creole spice

    2 tablespoons tomato paste

2 cloves of garlic

Creole Spice Mix:

2 tablespoons paprika

12 dried peri chili peppers

1 tablespoon salt

1 tablespoon freshly ground pepper

2 teaspoons dried thyme

2 teaspoons dried oregano

Directions:

Prepare the creole seasoning by blending all its ingredients
and preserve in a sealable jar.

Thread seitan and onion on the bamboo skewers in an
alternating pattern.

On a baking sheet, mix coconut milk with creole seasoning,
tomato paste and garlic.

Soak the skewers in the milk marinade for 2 hours.

Prepare and set up a grill over medium heat.

Grill the skewers for 7 minutes per side.

Serve.

Nutrition:

Calories: 407

Total Fat: 42g

Carbs: 13g

Net Carbs: 6g

Fiber: 1g

Protein: 4g

Mushroom Steaks

Preparation time: 10 minutes

Cooking time: 24 minutes

Servings: 04

Ingredients:

  1 tablespoon vegan butter

  1/2 cup vegetable broth

  1/2 small yellow onion, diced

  1 large garlic clove, minced

  3 tablespoons balsamic vinegar

  1 tablespoon mirin

  1/2 tablespoon soy sauce

  1/2 tablespoon tomato paste

  1 teaspoon dried thyme

  1/2 teaspoon dried basil

  A dash of ground black pepper

  2 large, whole portobello mushrooms

Directions:

Melt butter in a saucepan over medium heat and stir in half of the broth.

Bring to a simmer then add garlic and onion. Cook for 8 minutes.

Whisk the rest of the **Ingredients:** except the
mushrooms in a bowl.

Add this mixture to the onion in the pan and mix well.

Bring this filling to a simmer then remove from the
heat.

Clean the mushroom caps inside and out and divide
the filling between the mushrooms.

Place the mushrooms on a baking sheet and top them
with remaining sauce and broth.

Cover with foil then place it on a grill to smoke.

Cover the grill and broil for 16 minutes over indirect
heat.

Serve warm.

Nutrition:

Calories 379

Total Fat 29.7 g

Saturated Fat 18.6 g

Cholesterol 141 mg

Sodium 193 mg

Total Carbs 23.7g

Fiber 0.9 g

Sugar 1.3 g

Protein 5.2 g

Zucchini Boats with Garlic Sauce

Preparation time: 10 minutes

Cooking time: 10 minutes

Servings: 2

Ingredients:

> 1 zucchini
>
> 1 tablespoon olive oil
>
> Salt, to taste
>
> Black pepper, to taste

Filling:

> 1 cup organic walnuts
>
> 2 tablespoons olive oil
>
> 1/2 teaspoon smoked paprika
>
> 1/2 teaspoon ground cumin
>
> 1 pinch salt

Sauce:

> 1/2 cup cashews
>
> 1/2 cup water
>
> 2 teaspoons olive oil
>
> 2 teaspoons lemon juice
>
> 1 clove garlic
>
> 1/8teaspoon salt

Directions:

Cut the zucchini squash in half and scoop out some
flesh from the center to make boats.

Rub the zucchini boats with oil, salt, and black pepper.

Prepare and set up a grill over medium heat.

Grill the boats for 5 minutes per side.

In a blender, add all the filling **Ingredients:** and
blend them well.

Divide the filling between the zucchini boats.

Blend all of the sauce **Ingredients:** until it is lump
free.

Pour the sauce over the zucchini boats.

Serve.

Nutrition:

Calories 268

Total Fat 6 g

Saturated Fat 1.2 g

Cholesterol 351 mg

Sodium 103 mg

Total Carbs 12.8 g

Fiber 9.2 g

Sugar 2.9 g

Protein 7.2 g

Grilled Eggplant with Pecan Butter Sauce

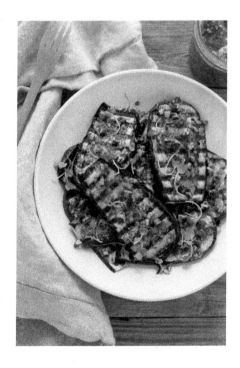

Preparation time: 10 minutes

Cooking time: 31 minutes

Servings: 02

Ingredients:

Marinated Eggplant:

1 eggplant, sliced

Salt to taste

4 tablespoons olive oil

1/4 teaspoon smoked paprika

1/4 teaspoon ground turmeric

Black Bean and Pecan Sauce:

1/3 cup vegetable broth

1/3 cup red wine

1/3 cup red wine vinegar

1 large shallot, chopped

1 teaspoon ground coriander

2 teaspoons minced cilantro

1/2 cup pecan pieces, toasted

2 roasted garlic cloves

4 small banana peppers, seeded, and diced

8 tablespoons vegan butter

1 tablespoon chives, chopped

1 (15.5 ounce) can black beans, rinsed and drained

Salt and black pepper to taste

1 teaspoon fresh lime juice

Directions:

In a saucepan, add broth, wine, vinegar, shallots, coriander, cilantro and garlic.

Cook while stirring for 20 minutes on a simmer.

Meanwhile blend butter with chives, pepper, and pecans in a blender.

Add this mixture to the broth along with salt, lime juice, black pepper, and beans.

Mix well and cook for 5 minutes.

Rub the eggplant with salt and spices.

Prepare and set up the grill over medium heat.

Grill the eggplant slices for 6 minutes per side.

Serve the eggplant with Prepared sauce.

Enjoy.

Nutrition:

Calories 201

Total Fat 32.2 g

Saturated Fat 2.4 g

Cholesterol 110 mg

Sodium 276 mg

Total Carbs 25 g

Fiber 0.9 g

Sugar 1.4 g

Protein 8.8 g

Sweet Potato Grilled Sandwich

Preparation time: 10 minutes

Cooking time: 12 minutes

Servings: 02

Ingredients:

> 1 small sweet potato, sliced
>
> 1/2 cup sweet bell peppers, sliced
>
> 1 cup canned black beans, roughly mashed
>
> 1/2 cup salsa
>
> 1 avocado, peeled and sliced
>
> 4 slices bread
>
> 1-2 tablespoons vegan butter

Directions:

Prepare and set up the grill over medium heat.

Grill the sweet potato slices for 5 minutes and the bell pepper slices for 3 minutes.

Spread each slice of bread liberally with butter.

On two of the bread slices, layer sweet potato slices, bell peppers, beans, salsa and avocado slices.

Place the other two slices of bread on top to make two sandwiches.

Cut them in half diagonally then grill the sandwiches for 1 minute per side.

Nutrition:

Calories 219

Total Fat 19.7 g

Saturated Fat 18.6 g

Cholesterol 141 mg

Sodium 193 mg

Total Carbs 23.7 g

Fiber 0.2 g

Sugar 1.3 g

Protein 5.2 g

Grilled Eggplant

Preparation time: 10 minutes

Cooking time: 10 minutes

Servings: 04

Ingredients:

2 tablespoons salt

1 cup water

3 medium eggplants, sliced

1/3 cup olive oil

Directions:

Mix water with salt in a bowl and soak eggplants for 10 minutes.

Drain the eggplant and leave them in a colander.

Pat them dry with a paper towel.

Prepare and set up the grill at medium heat.

Toss the eggplant slices in olive oil.

Grill them for 5 minutes per side.

Serve.

Nutrition:

Calories 248

Total Fat 15.7 g

Cholesterol 75 mg

Sodium 94 mg

Total Carbs 38.4 g

Fiber 0.3 g

Sugar 0.1 g

Protein 14.1 g

Grilled Portobello

Preparation time: 10 minutes

Cooking time: 8 minutes

Servings: 04

Ingredients:

  4 portobello mushrooms

  1/4 cup soy sauce

  1/4 cup tomato sauce

  2 tablespoons maple syrup

  1 tablespoon molasses

  2 tablespoons minced garlic

  1 tablespoon onion powder

  1 pinch salt and pepper

Directions:

  Mix all the **Ingredients:** except mushrooms in a
    bowl.

  Add mushrooms to this marinade and mix well to coat.

  Cover and marinate for 1 hour.

  Prepare and set up the grill at medium heat. Grease it
    with cooking spray.

  Grill the mushroom for 4 minutes per side.

  Serve.

Nutrition:

Calories 301

Total Fat 12.2 g

Cholesterol 110 mg

Sodium 276 mg

Total Carbs 12.5 g

Fiber 0.9 g

Sugar 1.4 g

Protein 8.8 g

Ginger Sweet Tofu

Preparation time: 10 minutes

Cooking time: 15 minutes

Servings: 04

Ingredients:

　　1/2 pound firm tofu, drained and diced

　　2 tablespoons peanut oil

　　1-inch piece ginger, sliced

　　1/3 pound bok choy, leaves separated

　　1 tablespoon shao sing rice wine

　　1 tablespoon rice vinegar

　　1/2 teaspoon dried chili flakes

Marinade:

　　1 tablespoon grated ginger

　　1 teaspoon dark soy sauce

　　2 tablespoons light soy sauce

　　1 tablespoon brown sugar

Directions:

Toss the tofu cubes with the marinade **Ingredients:**
　　and marinate for 15 minutes.

In a wok, add half of the oil and ginger, then sauté for
　　30 secs.

Toss in bok choy and cook for 2 minutes.

Add a splash of water and steam for 2 minutes.

Transfer the bok choy to a bowl.

Add remaining oil and tofu to the pan then sauté for 10 minutes.

Add the tofu to the bok choy.

Serve.

Nutrition:

Calories 119

Total Fat 14 g

Cholesterol 65 mg

Sodium 269 mg

Total Carbs 19 g

Fiber 4 g

Sugar 6 g

Protein 5g

Singapore Tofu

Preparation time: 10 minutes

Cooking time: 8 minutes

Servings: 04

Ingredients:

ounces fine rice noodles, boiled

4 ounces firm tofu, boiled

2 tablespoons sunflower oil

3 spring onions, shredded

1 small piece of ginger, chopped

1 red pepper, thinly sliced

ounces snap peas

ounces beansprouts

1 teaspoon tikka masala paste

2 teaspoons reduced-salt soy sauce

1 tablespoon sweet chili sauce

Chopped coriander and lime

Lime wedges, to serve

Directions:

In a wok, add 1 tablespoon oil and the tofu then sauté
for 5 minutes.

Transfer the sautéed tofu to a bowl.

Add more oil and the rest of the **Ingredients:** except noodles to the wok.

Stir fry for 3 minutes then add the tofu.

Toss well and then add noodles.

Mix and serve with lime wedges.

Nutrition:

Calories 231

Total Fat 20.1 g

Saturated Fat 2.4 g

Cholesterol 110 mg

Sodium 941 mg

Total Carbs 20.1 g

Fiber 0.9 g

Sugar 1.4 g

Protein 4.6 g

Wok Fried Broccoli

Preparation time: 10 minutes

Cooking time: 16 minutes

Servings: 02

Ingredients:

  3 ounces whole, blanched peanuts

  2 tablespoons olive oil

  1 banana shallot, sliced

  10 ounces broccoli, trimmed and cut into florets

  1/4 red pepper, julienned

  1/2 yellow pepper, julienned

  1 teaspoon soy sauce

Directions:

  Toast peanuts on a baking sheet for 15 minutes at 350
     degrees F.

  In a wok, add oil and shallots and sauté for 10 minutes.

  Toss in broccoli and peppers.

  Stir fry for 3 minutes then add the rest of the
     Ingredients:.

  Cook for 3 additional minutes and serve.

Nutrition:

Calories 361

Total Fat 16.3 g

Saturated Fat 4.9 g

Cholesterol 114 mg

Sodium 515 mg

Total Carbs 29.3 g

Fiber 0.1 g

Sugar 18.2 g

Protein 3.3 g

Broccoli & Brown Rice Satay

Preparation time: 10 minutes

Cooking time: 10 minutes

Servings: 4

Ingredients:

   6 trimmed broccoli florets, halved

   1-inch piece of ginger, shredded

   2 garlic cloves, shredded

   1 red onion, sliced

   1 roasted red pepper, cut into cubes

   2 teaspoons olive oil

   1 teaspoon mild chili powder

   1 tablespoon reduced salt soy sauce

   1 tablespoon maple syrup

   1 cup cooked brown rice

Directions:

Boil broccoli in water for 4 minutes then drain
   immediately.

In a pan add olive oil, ginger, onion, and garlic.

Stir fry for 2 minutes then add the rest of the
   Ingredients:.

Cook for 3 minutes then serve.

Nutrition:

Calories 205

Total Fat 22.7 g

Saturated Fat 6.1 g

Cholesterol 4 mg

Sodium 227 mg

Total Carbs 26.1 g

Fiber 1.4 g

Sugar 0.9 g

Protein 5.2 g

Sautéed Sesame Spinach

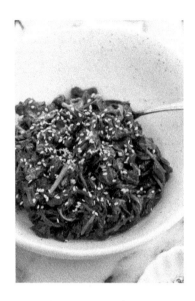

Preparation time: 1 hr. 10 minutes

Cooking time: 3 minutes

Servings: 04

Ingredients:

   1 tablespoon toasted sesame oil

   1/2 tablespoon soy sauce

   1/2 teaspoon toasted sesame seeds, crushed

   1/2 teaspoon rice vinegar

   1/2 teaspoon golden caster sugar

   1 garlic clove, grated

   8 ounces spinach, stem ends trimmed

Directions:

Sauté spinach in a pan until it is wilted.

Whisk the sesame oil, garlic, sugar, vinegar, sesame seeds, soy sauce and black pepper together in a bowl.

Stir in spinach and mix well.

Cover and refrigerate for 1 hour.

Serve.

Nutrition:

Calories 201

Total Fat 8.9 g

Cholesterol 57 mg

Sodium 340 mg

Total Carbs 24.7 g

Fiber 1.2 g

Sugar 1.3 g

Protein 15.3 g

Cajun Sweet Potatoes

Preparation Time: 5 minutes

Cooking Time: 30 minutes

Servings: 4

Ingredients:

- 2 pounds sweet potatoes
- 2 teaspoons extra-virgin olive oil
- ½ teaspoon ground cayenne pepper
- ½ teaspoon smoked paprika
- ½ teaspoon dried oregano
- ½ teaspoon dried thyme
- ½ teaspoon garlic powder
- ½ teaspoon salt (optional)

Directions:

1. Preheat the oven to 400°F. Line a baking sheet with parchment paper.
2. Wash the potatoes, pat dry, and cut into ¾-inch cubes. Transfer to a large bowl, and pour the olive oil over the potatoes.
3. In a small bowl, combine the cayenne, paprika, oregano, thyme, and garlic powder. Sprinkle the spices over the potatoes and combine until the potatoes are well coated. Spread the potatoes on the

prepared baking sheet in a single layer. Season with the salt (if using). Roast for 30 minutes, stirring the potatoes after 15 minutes.

4. Divide the potatoes evenly among 4 single-serving containers. Let cool completely before sealing.

Nutrition:

Calories: 219

Fat: 3g

Protein: 4g

Carbohydrates: 46g

Fiber: 7g

Sugar: 9g

Sodium: 125mg

Smoky Coleslaw

Preparation Time: 10 minutes

Cooking Time: 0 minute

Servings: 6

Ingredients:

1-pound shredded cabbage

1/3 cup vegan mayonnaise

¼ cup unseasoned rice vinegar

3 tablespoons plain vegan yogurt or plain soymilk

1 tablespoon vegan sugar

½ teaspoon salt

¼ teaspoon freshly ground black pepper

¼ teaspoon smoked paprika

¼ teaspoon chipotle powder

Directions:

Put the shredded cabbage in a large bowl. In a medium
bowl, whisk the mayonnaise, vinegar, yogurt, sugar,
salt, pepper, paprika, and chipotle powder.

Pour over the cabbage, and mix with a spoon or spatula and
until the cabbage shreds are coated. Divide the coleslaw
evenly among 6 single-serving containers. Seal the lids.

Nutrition:

Calories: 73

Fat: 4g

Protein: 1g

Carbohydrates: 8g

Fiber: 2g

Sugar: 5g

Sodium: 283mg

Mediterranean Hummus Pizza

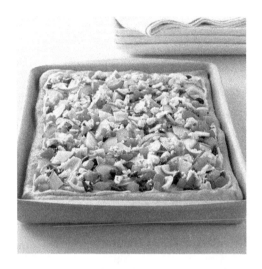

Preparation Time: 10 minutes

Cooking Time: 30 minutes

Servings: 2 pizzas

Ingredients:

½ zucchini, thinly sliced

½ red onion, thinly sliced

1 cup cherry tomatoes, halved

2 to 4 tablespoons pitted and chopped black olives

Pinch sea salt

Drizzle olive oil (optional)

2 prebaked pizza crusts

½ cup Classic Hummus

2 to 4 tablespoons Cheesy Sprinkle

Directions:

Preheat the oven to 400°F. Place the zucchini, onion, cherry tomatoes, and olives in a large bowl, sprinkle them with the sea salt, and toss them a bit. Drizzle with a bit of olive oil (if using), to seal in the flavor and keep them from drying out in the oven.

Lay the two crusts out on a large baking sheet. Spread half the hummus on each crust, and top with the veggie mixture and some Cheesy Sprinkle. Pop the pizzas in the oven for 20 to 30 minutes, or until the veggies are soft.

Nutrition:

Calories: 500; Total Fat: 25g

Carbs: 58g

Fiber: 12g

Protein:

Baked Brussels Sprouts

Preparation Time: 10 minutes

Cooking Time: 40 minutes

Servings: 4

Ingredients:

1-pound Brussels sprouts

2 teaspoons extra-virgin olive or canola oil

4 teaspoons minced garlic (about 4 cloves)

1 teaspoon dried oregano

½ teaspoon dried rosemary

½ teaspoon salt

¼ teaspoon freshly ground black pepper

1 tablespoon balsamic vinegar

Directions:

Preheat the oven to 400°F. Line a rimmed baking sheet with parchment paper. Trim and halve the Brussels sprouts. Transfer to a large bowl. Toss with the olive oil, garlic, oregano, rosemary, salt, and pepper to coat well.

Transfer to the prepared baking sheet. Bake for 35 to 40 minutes, shaking the pan occasionally to help with even browning, until crisp on the outside and tender on the inside. Remove from the oven and transfer to a large bowl. Stir in the balsamic vinegar, coating well.

Divide the Brussels sprouts evenly among 4 single-serving containers. Let cool before sealing the lids.

Nutrition:

Calories: 77

Fat: 3g

Protein: 4g

Carbohydrates: 12g

Fiber: 5g

Sugar: 3g

Sodium: 320mg

Minted Peas

Preparation Time: 5 minutes

Cooking Time: 5 minutes

Servings: 4

Ingredients:

1 tablespoon olive oil

4 cups peas, fresh or frozen (not canned)

½ teaspoon sea salt

freshly ground black pepper

3 tablespoons chopped fresh mint

Directions:

In a large sauté pan, heat the olive oil over medium-high
heat until hot. Add the peas and cook, about 5 minutes.
Remove the pan from heat. Stir in the salt, season with
pepper, and stir in the mint.
Serve hot.

Nutrition:

Calories: 77

Fat: 3g

Protein: 4g

Carbohydrates: 12g

Fiber: 5g

Sugar: 3g

Sodium: 320mg

Basic Baked Potatoes

Preparation Time: 5 minutes

Cooking Time: 60 minutes

Servings: 5

Ingredients:

> 5 medium Russet potatoes or a variety of potatoes, washed
> and patted dry
>
> 1 to 2 tablespoons extra-virgin olive oil
>
> ¼ teaspoon salt
>
> ¼ teaspoon freshly ground black pepper

Directions:

> Preheat the oven to 400°F. Pierce each potato several times
> with a fork or a knife. Brush the olive oil over the
> potatoes, then rub each with a pinch of the salt and a
> pinch of the pepper.
>
> Place the potatoes on a baking sheet and bake for 50 to 60
> minutes, until tender. Place the potatoes on a baking
> rack and cool completely. Transfer to an airtight
> container or 5 single-serving containers. Let cool before
> sealing the lids.

Nutrition:

Calories: 171

Fat: 3g

Protein: 4g

Carbohydrates: 34g

Fiber: 5g

Sugar: 3g

Sodium: 129mg

Glazed Curried Carrots

Preparation Time: 5 minutes

Cooking Time: 15 minutes

Servings: 6

Ingredients:

1-pound carrots, peeled and thinly sliced

2 tablespoons olive oil

2 tablespoons curry powder

2 tablespoons pure maple syrup

juice of ½ lemon

sea salt

freshly ground black pepper

Directions:

Place the carrots in a large pot and cover with water. Cook on medium-high heat until tender, about 10 minutes. Drain the carrots and return them to the pan over medium-low heat.

Stir in the olive oil, curry powder, maple syrup, and lemon juice. Cook, stirring constantly, until the liquid reduces, about 5 minutes. Season with salt and pepper and serve immediately.

Nutrition:

Calories: 171

Fat: 3g

Protein: 4g

Carbohydrates: 34g

Fiber: 5g

Sugar: 3g

Sodium: 129mg

Miso Spaghetti Squash

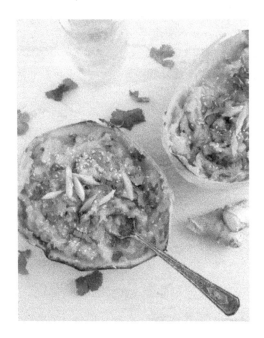

Preparation Time: 5 minutes

Cooking Time: 40 minutes

Servings: 4

Ingredients:

- 1 (3-pound) spaghetti squash
- 1 tablespoon hot water
- 1 tablespoon unseasoned rice vinegar
- 1 tablespoon white miso

Directions:

Preheat the oven to 400°F. Line a rimmed baking sheet with parchment paper. Halve the squash lengthwise and place, cut-side down, on the prepared baking sheet.

Bake for 35 to 40 minutes, until tender. Cool until the squash is easy to handle. With a fork, scrape out the flesh, which will be stringy, like spaghetti. Transfer to a large bowl. In a small bowl, combine the hot water, vinegar, and miso with a whisk or fork. Pour over the squash. Gently toss with tongs to coat the squash.

Divide the squash evenly among 4 single-serving containers. Let cool before sealing the lids.

Nutrition:

Calories: 117

Fat: 2g

Protein: 3g

Carbohydrates: 25g

Fiber: 0g

Sugar: 0g

Sodium: 218mg

Garlic and Herb Noodles

Preparation Time: 10 minutes

Cooking Time: 2 minutes

Servings: 4

Ingredients:

- 1 teaspoon extra-virgin olive oil or 2 tablespoons vegetable broth
- 1 teaspoon minced garlic (about 1 clove)
- 4 medium zucchinis, spiral
- ½ teaspoon dried basil
- ½ teaspoon dried oregano
- ¼ to ½ teaspoon red pepper flakes, to taste
- ¼ teaspoon salt (optional)
- ¼ teaspoon freshly ground black pepper

Directions:

In a large skillet over medium-high heat, heat the olive oil.

Add the garlic, zucchini, basil, oregano, red pepper flakes, salt (if using), and black pepper. Sauté for 1 to 2 minutes, until barely tender. Divide the noodles evenly among 4 storage containers. Let cool before sealing the lids.

Nutrition:

Calories: 44

Fat: 2g

Protein: 3g

Carbohydrates: 7g

Fiber: 2g

Sugar: 3g

Sodium: 20mg

Thai Roasted Broccoli

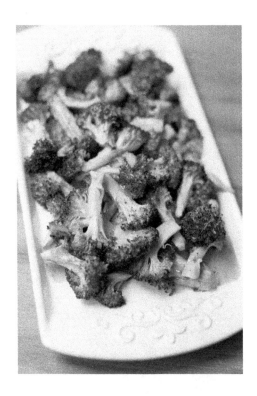

Preparation Time: 5 minutes

Cooking Time: 15 minutes

Servings: 4

Ingredients:

> 1 head broccoli, cut into florets
>
> 2 tablespoons olive oil
>
> 1 tablespoon soy sauce or gluten-free tamari

Directions:

Preheat the oven to 425°F. Line a baking sheet with
parchment paper. In a large bowl, combine the broccoli,
oil, and soy sauce. Toss well to combine.

Spread the broccoli on the prepared baking sheet. Roast for
10 minutes.

Toss the broccoli with a spatula and roast for an additional
5 minutes, or until the edges of the florets begin to
brown.

Nutrition:

Calories: 44

Fat: 2g

Protein: 3g

Carbohydrates: 7g

Fiber: 2g

Sugar: 3g

Sodium: 20mg

Coconut Curry Noodle

Preparation Time: 10 minutes

Cooking Time: 30 minutes

Servings: 4

Ingredients:

½ tablespoon oil

3 garlic cloves, minced

2 tablespoons lemongrass, minced

1 tablespoon fresh ginger, grated

2 tablespoons red curry paste

1 (14 oz) can coconut milk

1 tablespoon brown sugar

2 tablespoons soy sauce

2 tablespoons fresh lime juice

1 tablespoon hot chili paste

12 oz linguine

2 cups broccoli florets

1 cup carrots, shredded

1 cup edamame, shelled

1 red bell pepper, sliced

Directions:

Fill a suitably-sized pot with salted water and boil it on high heat.

Add pasta to the boiling water and cook until it is al dente then rinse under cold water.

Now place a medium-sized saucepan over medium heat and add oil.

Stir in ginger, garlic, and lemongrass, then sauté for 30 seconds.

Add coconut milk, soy sauce, curry paste, brown sugar, chili paste, and lime juice.

Stir this curry mixture for 10 minutes, or until it thickens.

Toss in carrots, broccoli, edamame, bell pepper, and cooked pasta.

Mix well, then serve warm.

Nutrition:

Calories: 44

Fat: 2g

Protein: 3g

Carbohydrates: 7g

Fiber: 2g

Sugar: 3g

Sodium: 20mg

Collard Green Pasta

Preparation Time: 10 minutes

Cooking Time: 20 minutes

Servings: 4

Ingredients

  2 tablespoons olive oil

  4 garlic cloves, minced

  8 oz whole wheat pasta

  ½ cup panko bread crumbs

  1 tablespoon nutritional yeast

  1 teaspoon red pepper flakes

  1 large bunch collard greens

  1 large lemon, zest and juiced

Directions:

Fill a suitable pot with salted water and boil it on high heat.

Add pasta to the boiling water and cook until it is al dente, then rinse under cold water.

Reserve ½ cup of the cooking liquid from the pasta.

Place a non-stick pan over medium heat and add 1 tablespoon olive oil.

Stir in half of the garlic, then sauté for 30 seconds.

Add breadcrumbs and sauté for approximately 5 minutes.

Toss in red pepper flakes and nutritional yeast then mix well.

Transfer the breadcrumbs mixture to a plate and clean the
pan.

Add the remaining tablespoon oil to the nonstick pan.

Stir in the garlic clove, salt, black pepper, and chard leaves.

Cook for 5 minutes until the leaves are wilted.

Add pasta along with the reserved pasta liquid.

Mix well, then add garlic crumbs, lemon juice, and zest.

Toss well, then serve warm.

Nutrition:

Calories: 45

Fat: 2.5g

Protein: 4g

Carbohydrates: 9g

Fiber: 4g

Sugar: 3g

Sodium: 20mg

Conclusion

In a nutshell, this cookbook offers you a world full of options to diversify your plant-based menu. People on this diet are usually seen struggling to choose between healthy food and flavor but, soon, they run out of the options. The selection of 250 recipes in this book is enough to adorn your dinner table with flavorsome, plant-based meals every day. Give each recipe a good read and try them out in the kitchen. You will experience tempting aromas and binding flavors every day.

The book is conceptualized with the idea of offering you a comprehensive view of a plant-based diet and how it can benefit the body. You may find the shift sudden, especially if you are a die-hard fan of non-vegetarian items. But you need not give up anything that you love. Eat everything in moderation.

The next step is to start experimenting with the different recipes in this book and see which ones are your favorites. Everyone has their favorite food, and you will surely find several of yours in this book. Start with breakfast and work your way through. You will be pleasantly surprised at how tasty a vegan meal really can be.

You will love reading this book, as it helps you to understand how revolutionary a plant-based diet can be. It will help you to make informed decisions as you move toward greater change for the greater good. What are you waiting for? Have you begun your journey on the path of the plant-based diet yet? If you haven't, do it now!

Now you have everything you need to get started making budget-friendly, healthy plant-based recipes. Just follow your basic shopping list and follow your meal plan to get started! It's easy to switch over to a plant-based diet if you have your meals planned out and temptation locked away. Don't forget to clean out your kitchen before starting, and you're sure to meet all your diet and health goals.

You need to plan if you are thinking about dieting. First, you can start slowly by just eating one meal a day, which is vegetarian and gradually increasing your number of vegetarian meals. Whenever you are struggling, ask your friend or family member to support you and keep you motivated. One important thing is also to be regularly accountable for not following the diet.

If dieting seems very important to you and you need to do it right, then it is recommended that you visit a professional such as a nutritionist or dietitian to discuss your dieting plan and optimizing it for the better.

No matter how much you want to lose weight, it is not advised that you decrease your calorie intake to an unhealthy level. Losing weight does not mean that you stop eating. It is done by carefully planning meals.

A plant-based diet is very easy once you get into it. At first, you will start to face a lot of difficulties, but if you start slowly, then you can face all the barriers and achieve your goal.

Swap out one unhealthy food item each week that you know is not helping you and put in its place one of the plant-based ingredients that you like. Then have some fun creating the many different recipes in this book. Find out what recipes you like the most so you can make them often and most of all; have some fun exploring all your recipe options.

Wish you good luck with the plant-based diet!

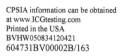

CPSIA information can be obtained
at www.ICGtesting.com
Printed in the USA
BVHW050834120421
604731BV00002B/163